Coconut Health Made

Simple

Coconut Oil Cures & Health Hacks to Lose Weight, Lower Cholesterol, Improve Your Memory, Hair, & Skin

By Anika Lindquist

Disclaimer

This book is presented solely for educational and entertainment purposes. For diagnosis or treatment of any medical problem, consult your own physician. The publisher and author are not responsible for any specific health or allergy needs that may require medical supervision and are not liable for any damages or negative consequences from any treatment, action, application or preparation, to any person reading or following the information in this book.

Although the author and publisher have made every effort to ensure that the information in this book was correct at press time, the author and publisher do not assume and hereby disclaim any liability to any party for any loss, damage, or disruption caused by errors or omissions, whether such errors or omissions result from negligence, accident, or any other cause.

Table of Contents

Introduction — **1**

Coconut Oil 101 — **3**

Coconut Oil for Weight Loss — **7**

Coconut Maple Granola — 13

Carrot-Apple Coconut Bran Muffins — 15

Rosemary-Garlic Seared Lamb Chops — 17

Chicken Lettuce Wraps — 19

Coconut-Berry Protein Shake — 21

Cajun-Style Okra — 23

Potato Salad — 24

Coconut Oil for Lowering Cholesterol — **27**

Coconut Oil for Slowing Aging — **31**

Top 5 Reasons to use Coconut Oil for Anti-Aging — 31

Coconut Oil for Reversing Alzheimer's Disease — **35**

What is Alzheimer's? — 35

Statistics — 36

Signs and Symptoms — 37

Treatment — 39

Alternative Medicine — 40

Coconut Oil for Beauty — **43**

Coconut Oil for the Skin — 44

Coconut Oil for the Body — 46

Coconut Oil for the Hair — 47

How to Incorporate Coconut Oil Into Your Life: A Daily Guide   **51**

Coconut Oil For Cooking   52

Smoothies, Soups, Hot Beverages, and Yogurts...Oh My!   53

Coconut Candy   53
    Coconut Chocolate   54

Toothpaste   56

Moisturizer   56

Scrubba Dub Dub, Coconut Oil is in the Tub!   56

Deodorant   57
    Dashing Deodorant   57

Oil Pulling   58

Hair Care   58

Guilt-free Mayo   58
    Smarter Mayo   59

Fight Yeast Infections   61

Sunscreen   61
    Simple Sunscreen   61

Energy Boost   62

Veins   62

Arthritis   63

Mosquito Bites, Poison Ivy, and Chicken Pox   63

Leather Softener   63

Throat Soother   63

Vapor Rub   63
    Vanquishing Vapor Rub   64

Hemorrhoid Help   64

Cold Sores   64

Acne Awareness   65

Heartburn and Nausea Soother   65

Warm Up   65

Conclusion   **67**

Other Books By Green Hills Press   **i**

Introduction

Now trending, coconut oil is being praised for its long-term weight loss support and endless health benefits. Unlike strict diets that force you into restricting certain foods and require you to purchase expensive foods that don't, in fact, meet your nutritional requirements, incorporating coconut oil into your everyday diet is simple and inexpensive.

With a recommended serving ranging from 1-4 tablespoons a day, adding in coconut oil does not demand that you totally change your diet. Instead, simply adding coconut oil into your morning cup of coffee or tea, replacing coconut oil for any fat you currently cook with, or tossing salad greens with a couple tablespoons of this versatile substance are just a few, easy ways to bring coconut oil into your life.

This book provides sound knowledge about the most significant benefits of coconut oil. Here you will find:

- an informational section about the basics of coconut oil
- how coconut oil aids in weight loss (recipes, too!)
- how coconut oil aids in lowering cholesterol
- how coconut oil slows aging
- how coconut oil can help reverse Alzheimer's
- how coconut oil promotes natural beauty
- a daily guide that shows you how to incorporate coconut oil into your life

Coconut oil, now classified as a "super food," increases metabolic rate, has multiple medicinal functions, curbs your appetite, lowers cholesterol, protects hair from becoming damaged and dry, boosts brain function, and can help you lose fat. Believe it or not, this list doesn't even represent half of coconut oil's benefits. Read on to find out more, and see for yourself how this tropical fruit oil can positively change your life.

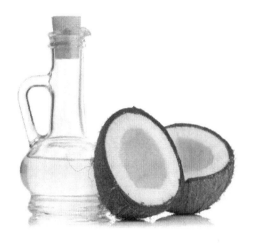

Coconut Oil 101

Coconut oil has been helping people lead healthier lives for thousands of years, both as a food and as a pharmaceutical substance. In Sanskrit medical documents dating back to 1500 BC, coconut oil was said to have healing properties for the spirit, body, and mind. Primarily made of medium-chain triglycerides, a healthy saturated fat, coconut oil can be used for cooking, for skin and hair care, for slowing the aging process, for lowering cholesterol, for weight loss, and for helping reverse Alzheimer's. In fact, during World War II, the water that came from the coconuts in the South Pacific was successfully used as a replacement for saline drip, and actually saved the lives of many soldiers.

Today, coconut oil is talked about on every health-related network, in every health- related magazine, in cookbooks, and by doctors, TV show hosts, and fitness instructors alike. Proven to be beneficial for overall immunity, to reducing hypertension, to help keep good cholesterol balanced, and to help reduce arterial injuries, coconut oil is an amazing substance. With its unique antibacterial, antiviral, anti-fungal, and anti-microbial properties, this tropical fruit oil plays an important role in today's overweight and disease-laden society. Heart disease, high blood pressure, and high cholesterol are only a few of the pressing health issues that we face nowadays. Coconut oil can be the start to a healthier, more fulfilling, stress and illness reduced life.

Although the benefits are clear and simple, when it comes to buying coconut oil, things can get a little tricky. With options such as organic, non-organic, refined, unrefined, virgin, extra virgin, cold-pressed, centrifuge extracted, and expeller-pressed, how do you know which coconut oil is worth the purchase? First and foremost: Read the labels. Any labels that mention the words coconut flakes, hydrogenated, or partially-hydrogenated, do not buy. These products have been chemically engineered, containing coarse solvents that have stripped the oil of its natural and beneficial properties. Organic, virgin, extra virgin, and cold-pressed are what you want to see on coconut oil labels. There is no difference between virgin and extra virgin coconut oil, as there is when comparing olive oils. All that means is that the oil is natural and unprocessed. Cold-pressed coconut oil is made from fresh, dried coconut flakes that have been kept at a low temperature. Although coconut flakes are included here, this type of coconut oil is considered raw, meaning that it possesses all of its nutrients. Along with all of these rich, organic qualities that coconut oil provides, it also gives a distinct taste to food, and a wonderfully tropical scent to any beauty products it's infused with.

From weight loss to Alzheimer's treatment, coconut oil is a fascinating and powerful substance. A diet consistent of managed amount of coconut oil reaps endless health benefits. Cooking with coconut oil is simple, as is making beauty products with a coconut oil base. This book will reveal to you some of the most significant perks of incorporating coconut oil into your life, and provide you with an everyday guide to make the transition of using coconut oil that much easier.

Coconut Oil for Weight Loss

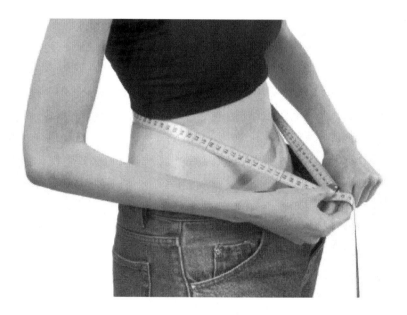

First it was South Beach, then Atkins, then a slimming club. Maybe the pounds came off in the beginning, but a few months later, you found yourself to have not only gained back the weight you lost, but to have gained back an additional ten or fifteen pounds. So what did you do? Picked up the latest trending diet book and started anew, promising yourself that this time you'll be better, you'll really be committed. Does this painful and discouraging cycle sound familiar? Are you tired of it? While it is important to stay health-conscious and ensure that your body receives the proper nutrients it needs to function properly, dieting just does not work for long-term health and weight loss results. In fact, dieting is unhealthy in that it forces your body to fluctuate far too much with weight loss and gain. That yo-yo dieting effect takes a huge toll on your body, potentially causing health issues, as opposed to promoting good health. So, if dieting is doomed to fail, what should you do? Let's consider going back to the unprocessed products that are so sadly overlooked in today's fast-paced, fast food-driven society. Let's take a look at coconut oil.

Contrary to popular belief, fat is essential for weight loss. Yes, that's right: Fat is essential for weight loss. And not just a little fat here and there, but a much more significant amount of fat is crucial for successful, long-term weight loss than is portrayed by the media. In fact, research has proven that a person who includes more fat in her diet generally eats less than a person who is consciously restricting fat. Fat satiates hunger, working as a natural appetite suppressant. Coconut oil contains fewer calories than any other fat. Replacing this for, say, olive oil when cooking will allow you to eat the same foods you love, while simultaneously consuming fewer calories. Not only will you consume fewer calories just because coconut oil has a lower caloric count than other fats, but it is also more satisfying than other fats, and will help you feel full quicker and longer. Well, just because coconut oil has fewer calories than other oils, and it works as an appetite suppressant, it's still very high in fat, so how will that aid in weight loss? Let's take a closer look.

Coconut oil is extremely unique in its properties, as well as its flavor! Instead of containing long-chain fatty acids, coconut oil contains medium-chain fatty acids. Okay...so what does this mean? It means that it is metabolized differently, more efficiently. It is thermogenic, meaning that eating it leads to an increase in energy disbursement, or fat burning. Essentially, coconut oil is great at speeding up your metabolism to help burn fat faster and longer. In fact, studies have shown that making coconut oil a regular part of your diet can help burn up to 120 extra calories per day. Simply adding in coconut oil to your diet will help you burn calories. It doesn't get much easier than that.

Coconut oil is specifically helpful when it comes to the reduction of belly fat. One study, conducted in 2009, focused on 40 women, aged 20-40, who were either given two tablespoons (30 grams) of coconut oil or soybean oil each day for 28 days. The results concluded that:

- Both groups of women lost about two pounds on average.

- Only the coconut oil group had a reported decrease in waist circumference, or belly fat. In fact, the soybean women had an increase in belly fat.

- The coconut oil group had a reported increase in good cholesterol levels, or HDL, while the soybean group had a decrease in HDL, and an increase in bad cholesterol levels, or LDL.

This study represents just one of many examples where coconut oil has been proven to reduce the harmful levels of belly fat. This dangerous abdominal fat, or visceral fat, is a leading factor is many diseases and illnesses, including, but not limited to:

- sleep apnea
- non-alcoholic fatty liver disease
- type two diabetes
- high blood pressure
- colon cancer
- coronary heart disease
- metabolic syndrome

Coconut oil, as it acts as a natural appetite suppressant and contains fewer calories than other fats, can help you kiss this cruel fat goodbye. In order to do this successfully, use coconut oil to replace the fats that you have been cooking with. This is not to say that you can double up on coconut oil, but using an appropriate amount is key for long-term weight loss and health goals. So, what is an appropriate amount of coconut oil? Let's take a look at some guidelines and a few recipes to get you started on dropping those extra pounds and improving your overall health.

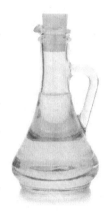

For most women, at least one tablespoon of coconut oil taken daily is the recommended amount. While you can cook vegetables, eggs, and meat with coconut oil, there are other ways of getting it into your system. For example, mix in one tablespoon of liquid coconut oil (simply melt it in the microwave) with your oatmeal or yogurt. Stir in a tablespoon with your coffee or tea for a hint of tropical flavoring. For a snack, spread a little coconut oil over crackers or bread. Any way that you choose is fine, as long as you don't go overboard. Again, one to two tablespoons a day, in place of another fat, is what is most commonly suggested. If you have other questions or concerns, feel free to consult your doctor for further guidance.

Coconut Maple Granola

Serves 12

Time involved: 5-10

minutes prepping; 25-30

minutes cooking

Equipment needed:

large mixing bowl; large

rimmed baking sheet

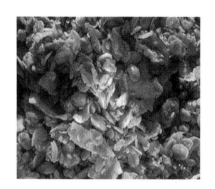

3 cups rolled oats

1/4 cup unsweetened coconut flakes

1/2 cup unsweetened coconut shreds

3/4 cups raw almonds

1/3 cup virgin coconut oil (melted)

1/8 cup brown sugar

1/4 cup maple syrup

1/2 tsp salt

1. Preheat the oven to 350°F.
2. Combine oats, almonds, coconut oil, both types of coconut, and maple syrup into a large bowl. Stir well. Then add in the brown sugar, and stir. Season with salt.

3. Over a large rimmed baking sheet, spread the granola. Bake for 25-30 minutes, stirring the granola every 10 minutes.

4. Once baked, let the granola cool completely before serving.

Nutrition Facts (per serving):

Calories 187   Fat 10.3g

Carbs 21g   Protein 4g

Carrot-Apple Coconut Bran Muffins

Serves 12-15

Time involved: 5-10

minutes prepping; 20-25

minutes cooking

Equipment needed:

muffin tin; 2 mixing

bowls

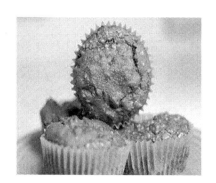

1 cup unprocessed oat bran

1 cup whole wheat flour

1/2 tsp salt

1 1/4 tsp baking soda

2 eggs

2 tbsp molasses

6 tbsp honey

1/4 cup virgin coconut oil (melted)

3/4 cup whole milk

1 cup carrots (grated finely)

1/2 cup shredded coconut

1/2 cup Granny Smith apples (diced)

1/2 cup walnuts

1. Preheat oven to 350°F.

2. In a mixing bowl, combine all of the dry ingredients.

3. In a separate bowl, beat the eggs. Then add in the honey, molasses, milk, and oil (make sure it's in that order), and whisk.

4. In the dry ingredients, make a small well, and pour the liquid ingredients in. Whisk until well combined. Add in the apples, shredded coconut, shredded carrots, and walnuts.

5. In a paper-lined or greased muffin pan, pour in the batter. Fill each cup about 3/4 of the way full. Bake for 20-25 minutes, or until an inserted toothpick comes out clean.

Nutrition Facts (per serving):

Calories 175   Fat 5.6g

Carbs 23.4g   Protein 4.2g

Rosemary-Garlic Seared Lamb Chops

Serves 3-4

Time involved: 10 minutes

prepping; 20-25 minutes

cooking

Equipment needed: food

processor; 1 small skillet; 1

oven-safe skillet

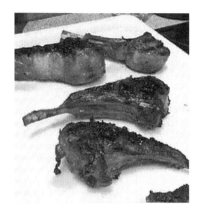

6 lamb rib chops

3 garlic cloves (peeled, chopped)

1/4 cup rosemary (remove leaves from stems)

2 tbsp coconut oil

Sea salt and black pepper to taste

1. Preheat oven to 400°F.
2. Pulse the garlic and rosemary in a food processor until minced finely.
3. Sauté the garlic and rosemary in 1 tbsp of coconut oil in a small skillet. Set aside when lightly browned.

4. Rinse the lamb chops under cool water, and pat dry with a paper towel. To your liking, sprinkle each chop with sea salt and black pepper.

5. Heat 1 tbsp of coconut oil in a oven-safe skillet over medium heat. Sear each chop for 2 minutes on each side.

6. Top the chops with the sautéed garlic and rosemary, and place in the oven. Bake for 2 minutes. Serve immediately.

Nutrition Facts (per serving):

Calories 260   Fat 15.3g

Carbs 3.5g   Protein 26.6g

Chicken Lettuce Wraps

Serves 4

Time involved: 5-10 minutes prepping; 20 minutes cooking

Equipment needed: 1 skillet

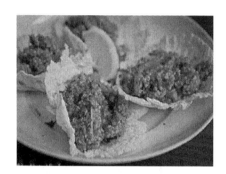

3 boneless chicken breasts (cubed)

2 tbsp virgin coconut oil

3 cloves of garlic (diced finely)

1 in piece of ginger (diced)

1 green bell pepper (diced)

1/2 tsp crushed red pepper

4 green onions (sliced)

3/4 cup button mushrooms (diced)

1 head of lettuce (leaves detached)

2 tbsp tamari

Sea salt and black pepper to taste

1. In a skillet, heat the coconut oil. Add in the garlic and ginger, and sauté for a few minutes or until lightly browned.

2. Add in the chicken and crushed pepper to the skillet. Cook until the chicken is cooked through, or for 5-7 minutes.

3. Then add in the mushrooms and bell pepper, and cook for a few additional minutes.

4. Lastly, add in the tamari with the green onions. Season with sea salt and black pepper. Serve over a few lettuce leaves.

Nutrition Facts (per serving):

Calories 222   Fat 4.3g

Carbs 7.1g   Protein 39g

There are hundreds of more recipes like these just waiting to be discovered. From breakfast to dessert, coconut oil can replace a fat in just about any meal or snack. Don't hesitate to substitute coconut oil in any and all of your favorite recipes.

Coconut-Berry Protein Shake

Serves 2

Time involved: Under 5 minutes total

Equipment needed: Blender

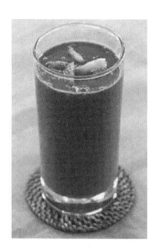

1 cup of your favorite berries

1 cup coconut milk (full fat)

1 tbsp coconut oil

1 tbsp almond butter

1 egg

1 tbsp flaxseed

1/3 tsp sea salt

1. In a blender, place the berries, coconut milk, and almond butter. Blend on high until thoroughly mixed.
2. Then blend in the oil, flaxseed, and salt. Blend the eggs in last, but only for a few seconds.
3. Pour into a glass and enjoy immediately.

Nutrition Facts (per serving):

Calories 456   Fat 43.3g

Carbs 13.8g   Protein 8.7g

Cajun-Style Okra

Serves 4

Time involved: 5 minutes prepping; 10 minutes cooking

Equipment needed: 1 large skillet

1 lb okra (sliced 1/4 in. thick)

2 tbsp coconut oil

1/2 tsp dried thyme

1/2 tsp dried oregano

1 onion (sliced thinly)

1 hot pepper

1. Melt the coconut oil over medium heat in a large skillet.
2. Add in the pepper, onion, and herbs, and sauté until the onions have softened.
3. Add in the okra and cook for about 5 minutes, stirring occasionally.

Nutrition Facts (per serving):

Calories 109   Fat 7g

Carbs 11.2g   Protein 2.4g

Potato Salad

Serves 6

Time involved: 5 minutes prepping; 15 minutes cooking

Equipment needed: 1 stock pot; 1 mixing bowl

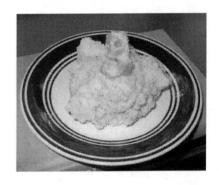

2 lbs new potatoes (cut into quarters)

1 tbsp Dijon mustard

1 tbsp rosemary

1/3 cup coconut oil

1 tsp salt

1. Cover potatoes with water in a stock pot. Bring the potatoes to a boil on high heat, then reduce to a simmer. Cook for 10 minutes.
2. As the potatoes boil, mix together the coconut oil, mustard, salt, and rosemary in bowl.
3. Once the potatoes have been cooked and drained, carefully toss the sauce mixture with the potatoes until well covered. Serve warm.

Nutrition Facts (per serving):

Calories 212   Fat 12.4g

Carbs 24.2g   Protein 2.7g

Coconut Oil for Lowering Cholesterol

Among its many health benefits, coconut oil lends a helping hand in lowering bad (LDL) cholesterol. According to a group of co-medical directors of Inner Source Health in New York, "Coconut oil lowers cholesterol

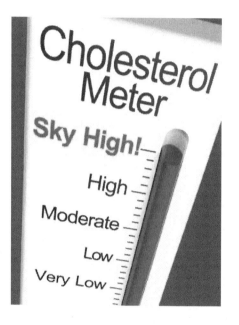

by promoting its conversion to pregnenolone, a molecule that is a precursor to many of the hormones our bodies need. Coconut can help restore thyroid function. When the thyroid does not function optimally, it can contribute to higher levels of bad cholesterol." Coconut oil helps to keep a more balanced cholesterol ratio. While most people get caught up on their overall cholesterol level, Dr. Bruce Fife says that what is most important is the ratio. "While coconut oil does not reduce overall cholesterol as effectively as polyunsaturated oils do," says Fife, "it has a greater effect on HDL" -- good cholesterol. Fife continues to note that, "When HDL levels are evaluated, coconut oil reduces risk of heart disease more than soybean, canola, safflower, or any other vegetable oil typically recommended as 'heart healthy.'" In conclusion, "coconut oil is the best oil you can use to protect yourself from heart disease," says Fife.

Incorporating coconut oil into a balanced diet reaps long-term health benefits. According to Ray Peat, PhD, "Coconut oil slightly lowers cholesterol level, which is exactly what is expected when a dietary change raises thyroid function. This same increase in thyroid function and metabolic rate explains why people and animals that regularly eat coconut oil are lean, and remarkably free of heart disease and cancer." Coconut oil's natural properties of medium-chain fatty acids allow it to be such a useful tool when it comes to lowering cholesterol. Since these acids increase the rate of fat burning, or metabolic rate, HDL is boosted, while LDL is lowered.

In order to successfully lower your bad cholesterol and raise your good cholesterol, NaturalNews.com recommends that you should consume three to four tablespoons of natural, unprocessed coconut oil daily. Even if you don't like to cook, there are many simple ways to incorporate coconut oil into your everyday routine. For example:

- Blend 1-2 tablespoons of coconut oil into your favorite fruit smoothie mix.
- Stir in 1 tablespoon of coconut oil to your morning oatmeal, or yogurt.
- Mix salad greens with 1-3 tablespoons of coconut oil.
- Spread 1-2 tablespoons of coconut oil over toast or crackers.
- Take 1 coconut oil supplement with a meal.

Lowering your cholesterol will give you more energy, and help prevent heart-related diseases and conditions. It's not difficult to include coconut oil in your diet, but it is up to you to make the change.

Coconut Oil for Slowing Aging

Coconut oil, in its pure and natural form, is one of the safest anti-aging products available. Aging, the formation of wrinkles and sagging, happens when there is a buildup of free radicals -- an uncharged molecule having an unpaired valence electron -- within the skin. These free radicals cause damage to the connective tissues in the skin, which is manifested as wrinkles and sagging. In order to keep that youthful elasticity in your skin, you need to maintain a moisturizing regimen. Organic coconut oil contains many antioxidants that help slow down the aging process by aiding the connective tissues to keep their elasticity.

Top 5 Reasons to use Coconut Oil for Anti-Aging

Collagen production: Coconut oil naturally increases the production of collagen, the substance that keeps skin looking tight and smooth.

Moisture: Moisturized skin is less prone to wrinkles, and coconut oil is an excellent source of moisturizer. In fact, many over-the-counter lotion and skin care products contain coconut oil, but pure organic coconut oil is vastly superior to chemically engineered products.

Cook the years away: Using coconut oil to cook with will keep your body young from the inside out.

Oh, sugar: Sugar has been proven to aggravate aging, eating away at the healthy proteins in our skin that keeps it looking springy and youthful. Adding coconut oil into your diet can help curb your appetite, essentially curbing your sugar cravings.

Immunity insurance: Coconut oil is used for a variety of medicinal purposes, one of which is to strengthen your immune system. A strong immune system will make illnesses less frequent, and easier to fight off.

While looking young tends to take precedence over keeping our organs and internal selves young in today's society, it is critically important that we don't overlook the immunity benefits that coconut oil provides. Aging is a process that starts from within, so if you desperately desire to look young on the outside, you need to work first from the inside.

Several studies have shown that a daily intake of coconut oil can significantly help our bodies build resistance to both bacteria and viruses. As we age and our bodies become weaker, even something as minor as the common cold presents us with more of a threat. Coconut, in its various forms, is rich with medium-chain saturated fats that have crucial antimicrobial properties, meaning it helps kill harmful fungi, parasites, bacteria, and viruses. Some illnesses that coconut has been known to treat are giardia, lice, throat infections, influenza, tapeworms, urinary tract infections, gonorrhea, herpes, and bronchitis. Simply adding a teaspoon of coconut oil to your morning coffee or tea can help you protect your body and strengthen your immune system. Stay young from within, and your external features will radiate youth.

Coconut Oil for Reversing Alzheimer's Disease

What is Alzheimer's?

Alzheimer's disease is a form of dementia -- a loss of brain function that occurs with some diseases -- that slowly gets worse over time. It affects behavior, thinking, and memory. Those affected by Alzheimer's 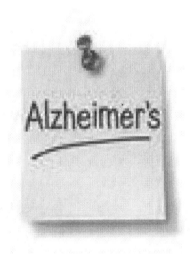 are more likely to be older, have a close blood relative with the disease, and be genetically predisposed. Other factors such as being female, having a history of head trauma, and having a history of high blood pressure may also increase your risk of developing AD. There are two types of Alzheimer's, early onset and late onset. Early onset is much less common than late onset, where symptoms begin before the age of 60. The loss of brain function occurs at a more rapid pace with early onset, and it usually runs in families. Late onset, or the most common type of AD, occurs in those over 60 years old, and it may run in some families.

Statistics

The following statistics, as adapted from the Alzheimer's Foundation of America, are geared to give an overview of the disease and its impact on today's society.

- An estimate shows that nearly 5.1 million Americans are Alzheimer's candidates.

- The aging population is experiencing a frequency in rates of Alzheimer's Disease.

- According to research from the National Institute of Aging, the likelihood of someone developing Alzheimer's Disease doubles every five years past the age of 65.

- An estimate shows that about half a million Americans younger than 65 show some signs of dementia, including Alzheimer's disease.

- An estimate shows that 1-4 family members serve as caregivers for each individual suffering from Alzheimer's disease.

Signs and Symptoms

Generally, Alzheimer's symptoms revolve around a difficulty with a handful of areas of mental function. These include:

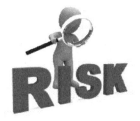

- Language
- Memory
- Emotional behavior
- Personality
- Perception
- Cognitive skills (judgment and thinking)

Initially, AD first surfaces as forgetfulness. This doesn't have to be major forgetfulness, but just minor things. For example, forgetting where you put your glasses, forgetting certain words or places, forgetting to pay a bill. However, not all minor forgetfulness leads to AD, some is due to the normal aging process. More serious symptoms to be aware of are:

- Difficulty to perform tasks that use some thought, but used to come easily. This includes, playing card games, learning new information, and writing a check

- Having trouble recalling the name of everyday/familiar objects

- Misplacing things

- Flat mood, or a significant loss of interest in activities that used to be regularly enjoyed

- Changes in personality and social awkwardness

As Alzheimer's continues to develop, and symptoms become more obvious and frequent, there are other patterns to look out for. They include:

- Depression

- Agitation

- Delusions

- Waking up at night, or other changes in sleep patterns
- Difficulty getting dressed/choosing appropriate clothes
- Difficulty preparing meals
- Difficulty writing
- Difficulty reading
- Forgetting events in your life history
- Loss of self-awareness
- Poor judgment (could lead you to situations that present danger)
- Difficulty feeding yourself
- Difficulty bathing

Treatment

Unfortunately, there is no cure for Alzheimer's disease. Some prescription drugs and over-the-counter supplements have been shown to help ease symptoms. Most people who suffer undergo treatment to help:

- Manage symptoms that deal with behavior, sleep disturbance, and confusion
- Slow the disease's progression
- Better perform everyday activities by changing the home environment
- Get support from loved ones and/or educated caregivers

While these methods can be helpful, the pace of Alzheimer's affects each person differently, so some options may be more beneficial than others. Traditionally, if AD develops rapidly, it is much more likely to worsen at the same speed.

Alternative Medicine

Treating Alzheimer's is very expensive. In the US, the cost of treatment has been estimated at $148 billion. Prescription medicines, private caregivers, assisted living homes, and nursing homes are not always accessible for families struggling in today's economy. In fact, the latest research proves that common drugs used to treat Alzheimer's -- like Aricept -- have yielded unimpressive or no results, and only complicate matters for the individual with undesirable side effects. Fortunately, there have been other, more affordable resources to help with Alzheimer's, and one of the leading substances is coconut oil.

With Alzheimer's, specific brain cells usually have a hard time accessing and using glucose -- mainly used from carbohydrates included in the diet -- the brain's main source of fuel. Ironically, an alternative source of brain energy is stored in ketones, which are naturally produced in the brain when the body is deprived of carbohydrates. Since it's not very appealing to cut carbohydrates out of one's diet, research shows that ketones can also be helped produced by consuming oils high in medium chain fatty acids -- like coconut oil.

Research shows that an added dose of 20 grams (about 4 teaspoons) of coconut oil into your daily diet can not only protect against prevalence of Alzheimer's, but may actually work to reverse it. Posted on the Alliance for Natural Health's webpage is a testimonial about Dr. Mary Newport's husband who suffered from

Alzheimer's for years on prescription medicine. When her husband started taking coconut oil just twice a day, his symptoms gradually reversed themselves. He was "able to run again, his reading comprehension [improved] dramatically, and his short-term memory [improved] -- he often [brought] up events that happened days to weeks earlier and [relayed] telephone conversations with accurate detail. A recent MRI shows that the brain atrophy [had] been completely halted."

Although coconut oil cannot cure Alzheimer's disease, as there is no cure, it has been proven to slow the progression of the disease for those experiencing early symptoms, as well as reverse the disease for those for whom it has already developed. Simply adding a couple tablespoons a day to your diet can help with this miraculous process. Cook your vegetables and/or meat in coconut oil. Stir some in to a cup of morning coffee or tea. Blend some in with your favorite fruit smoothie. These easy options can help you and your loved ones fight the battle of Alzheimer's.

Coconut Oil for Beauty

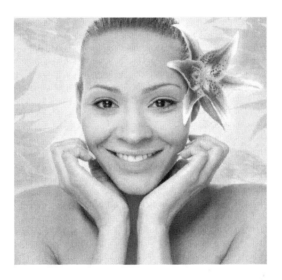

Coconut oil, found in many natural beauty products, is naturally antibacterial and antifungal and a terrific moisturizer. It can penetrate hair more effectively than other oils. Not to mention that it smells like heaven. Celebrities such as Victoria's Secret model Miranda Kerr, Demi Moore, and Madonna all advocate for coconut oil's superior qualities. While coconut oil can be consumed, no ingestion is necessary to yield the benefits. The following is a list of 21, do-it-yourself beauty products for skin, body, and hair care. All you will need is virgin coconut oil to let your radiance shine.

Coconut Oil for the Skin

A safe and effective solution that helps prevent the drying and cracking of skin, coconut oil also helps in hindering the occurrence of wrinkles and sagging. It also helps treat eczema, dermatitis, psoriasis, and a variety of other skin infections, as well as premature aging.

1. **Face mask**: Want the softest skin possible? Simple. Combine equal parts of coconut oil and honey, and mix well. Apply the mixture onto your face for 10 minutes, and immediately notice the moisture and softness that has been restored.

2. **Face scrub**: For those stubborn imperfections, try mixing equal amounts of coconut oil and baking soda for a refreshing scrub.

3. **Lip balm**: Easy as (coconut) pie. Simply finger on some plain, virgin coconut oil onto your lips for extreme moisture.

4. **Makeup remover**: Remove all that dirt from your face by simply rubbing coconut oil into your skin. Wipe away with a wash cloth, and rinse your face well. Not only will the makeup be gone, but your skin will feel incredible soft and smooth.

5. **Acne**: Mix 1 tbsp of coconut oil with 1 tbsp of nutmeg. Apply to blemishes for 10-15 minutes, then wash off. Do this up to two times a day.

6. **Age spots**: Apply coconut oil directly to age spots and watch as they fade over time. The properties in coconut oil help prevent free-radical formation.

7. **Shaving cream**: Replace your typical shaving cream with coconut oil, and feel the difference in smoothness.

Coconut Oil for the Body

Coconut oil has healing properties that have been proven to heal ease the symptoms of topical infections. Along with being an excellent moisturizer, coconut oil also aids in restoring damaged tissue, such as with bruises. Applying coconut oil to bruises will expedite the healing process by quickly mending the injured tissue.

1. **Exfoliating scrub**: Combine equal parts of coconut oil with sea salt to create a moisturizing scrub.

2. **Penetrating moisturizer**: Mix together equal parts of coconut oil and olive oil to make the best lotion you've ever tried!

3. **Cellulite crusher**: Combine 1 cup of coconut oil, 1 cup of jojoba oil, 1 tbsp cyprus oil, 1 tbsp lavender oil, and 1 tbsp of juniper oil. Massage into the cellulite areas overnight. Repeat nightly.

4. **Shiny new you**: Rub coconut oil over your whole body to create a beautiful, head-turning glow to your skin.

5. **Foot fixer**: Do the words cracked and dry describe your feet? Rub some coconut oil over the dry areas and rub with a pumice stone. Then rub in a little more coconut oil, put on a pair of cozy socks, and let the magic work overnight.

6. **New nails**: Massage a little coconut oil into your cuticles and nails to help build strength.

7. **Eczema**: Apply coconut oil to the affected area 3-4 times a day. You don't need a heavy coating, just a light one will do.

Coconut Oil for the Hair

Serving as a natural nutrient for your hair, coconut oil helps grow your hair healthfully, keep it shiny, and restore essential proteins that keep your hair strong. It also aids in the re-growth of damaged hair, as well as protecting hair from lice.

1. **Conditioner:** Massage a few drops (about 1 tsp) of coconut oil into wet or dry hair, and leave in overnight. Shampoo the next morning and feel the silky goodness.

2. **Deep conditioner**: Use the flesh from half an avocado and 4 tbsp of coconut oil, and mix well in a bowl. Massage the paste into damp hair, and comb through to distribute evenly. Leave in for 20 minutes and then rinse out with shampoo.

3. **Hair strengthener**: Heat 3 tbsp of coconut oil in the microwave, and the let cool a bit. Beat an egg in with the heated coconut oil, put the mixture in a plastic bag, and wrap the bag around your hair for an hour. Wash out with shampoo.

4. **Frizzy fix**: Take a tiny, pea-sized, portion of coconut oil and rub it in between your palms. For straight hair, run your hands over your hair and smooth away the frizz. For curly hair, run your fingers/palms through your hair and squeeze.

5. **Dandruff**: Massage coconut oil into your scalp and hair for 5 minutes. Let sit for 30-60 minutes. Shampoo and rinse.

6. **Premature grays**: Grind a handful of curry leaves with a little water as to make a paste. Mix the paste with 2 cups of coconut oil, and heat the mixture until all of the moisture has evaporated.

Store in a bottle after is cools. Every two weeks, massage the mixtures into your hair 2-3 times. Leave it in overnight for more effective results.

7. **Gummy situation**: If you happen to find yourself (or your child) with gum caught in your hair, simply apply coconut oil to the problem area, wait an hour, and the gum will slide right out.

Along with acting as a beauty agent, coconut oil has some pretty effective and helpful uses for your wellbeing. When you feel better about yourself, when your confidence is up, that is when your beauty shines through. Let coconut oil help you discover your pure, natural beauty.

Hot Flashes: Put a healthy portion of coconut oil on your scalp and hair before going to bed. Lay a towel over your pillow, and let the coconut oil soak in overnight. This will help cool your hot flashes. Simply rinse the oil out in the morning.

Mood Booster: For a relaxing, peaceful massage oil, melt 1 cup of coconut oil over the stove, and add in a handful of lavender, rosemary, or basil. Let simmer for 30 minutes low heat, making sure it doesn't boil, and stir often. Store in a jar, and place in the refrigerator. When you're feeling down, massage a bit of the mix on your body (maybe if you're sore or achy) to help ease your pain.

Time of the Month: Apply this blend to your abdomen when experiencing menstrual cramps: Combine 1/2 cup of coconut oil, 1 tsp lavender oil, 1 tsp cyprus oil, and 1 tsp chamomile oil. Mix well.

How to Incorporate Coconut Oil Into Your Life: A Daily Guide

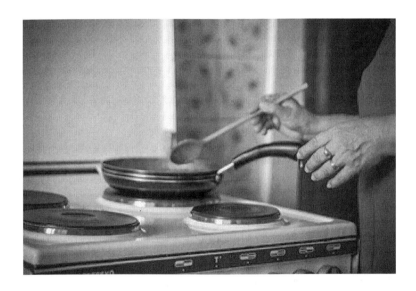

At this point in the book, you have read up on the incredible benefits of coconut oil. You have learned that it strengthens your immune system, revs up your metabolism, acts as an appetite suppressant, kills fungi and bacteria, supports thyroid function, helps reverse Alzheimer's disease, lowers bad cholesterol, raises good cholesterol, aids in preventing wrinkles and saggy skin, and can improve skin and hair health. You have also picked up a few tips and recipes about incorporating coconut oil into your diet and lifestyle. What follows is a simple, complete list of ways to include coconut oil into your daily routine. There is no reason not to integrate this fantastic substance into your life!

Coconut Oil For Cooking

This is probably the most common way people incorporate coconut oil into their everyday lives. It's simple -- replace whatever cooking oil you have been using with coconut oil, and experience all of the health benefits it has to offer, along with a brilliant, tropical flavor. From baked goods to eggs, there is always room for coconut oil in your diet. Here's a list to get you started:

- Before roasting, toss vegetables in coconut oil.
- Learn to love raw desserts that commonly feature coconut oil.
- Use as butter for spreading over bread, toast, crackers.
- Make homemade salad dressing, and use coconut oil as the base.

- Just eat it! Consume 1-2 tablespoons of coconut oil.

Smoothies, Soups, Hot Beverages, and Yogurts...Oh My!

Along with cooking, adding coconut oil into your favorites is always an option. Try adding 1 tablespoon of melted coconut oil in with your favorite smoothie blend and yogurts. A half a tablespoon in hot chocolate or chicken soup will melt right in; just make sure to stir a bit.

Coconut Candy

This is probably the tastiest way to include coconut oil in your life. Here's a recipe for chocolate bars with coconut oil!

On the following page is a recipe for coconut candy. Enjoy!

Coconut Chocolate

Serves 10

Time involved: 5 minutes prepping; 5-10 minutes cooking; 2-4 hours refrigerating

Equipment needed: 1 small saucepan; 1 mixing bowl; 1 cookie sheet; parchment paper

2/3 cup coconut oil

2/3 cup cocoa powder

1/2 tsp vanilla extract

1/3 cup + 1 tbsp maple syrup

1/2 tsp salt

1. In a small saucepan over low heat, warm the coconut oil. Once melted, add in the remaining ingredients.
2. Stir until the ingredients are combined well. Then pour the mixture over a cookie sheet lined with parchment paper.
3. Put the chocolate-covered cookie sheet in the refrigerator for 2-4 hours, or until the chocolate has set hard.

4. Once the chocolate is completely hard, break it up into pieces. You can store the chocolate in a sealed container, and keep it refrigerated.

Nutrition Facts (per serving):

Calories 171   Fat 15.3g

Carbs 11.6g   Protein 1g

Toothpaste

Although this may sound strange, coconut oil is an excellent substance for cleaning your teeth and mouth. Since coconut oil kills bacteria, and your mouth is prone to collecting such, mixing coconut oil with baking soda and sea salt makes for a very effective toothpaste. If you're not into going full-out coconut oil, try rubbing a little on your toothbrush before applying your regular paste.

Moisturizer

For super soft and smooth skin, coconut oil will outdo any fancy store-bought lotion any day. Apply to wherever is needed, especially if you are experiencing dry, flaky, or itchy skin. Also, coconut oil has been known to help clear up diaper rash and eczema, more serious skin issues.

Scrubba Dub Dub, Coconut Oil is in the Tub!

By just adding a teaspoon of coconut oil into your bath water, your body and sense of smell will become relaxed. To make a scrub and enhance this sensation, simply mix equal parts of coconut oil and sea salt to create an exfoliating blend that will leave your body feeling and looking refreshed.

Deodorant

While you can directly apply coconut oil to your underarms as a deodorant, check out this homemade recipe for a more well-rounded remedy:

Dashing Deodorant

1/4 cup arrowroot powder

1/4 cup baking soda

4 tbsp coconut oil (soft, at room temperature)

1/4 tsp tea tree oil

1. In a bowl, mix all ingredients until they're combined well. Store the blend in an airtight container, or pour it into empty deodorant containers.
2. *For sensitive skin, decrease the baking soda by 2 tbsp, and increase the arrowroot powder by 2 tbsp.

Oil Pulling

Oil what? Oil pulling, which dates back thousands of years to Ayurvedic medicine, works as a cleansing process to rid the body of bacteria and sinuses! It's simple; just rinse your mouth out with liquid coconut oil. If you can, swish it around your mouth for 5 minutes. It may sound gross, but it has been proven, time and time again, to get rid of head colds, headaches, and help with sinus relief.

Hair Care

Massage a tablespoon of virgin coconut oil into your hair and scalp, and let it sit for at least an hour. Wash your hair. Do this up to three times each week for nourishment and to prevent hair from breaking and/or becoming dry.

Guilt-free Mayo

Big mayo lover? Check out this healthy, alternative mayonnaise recipe to keep your taste buds and waistline happy.

Smarter Mayo

Serves 20

Time involved: 5 minutes total

Equipment needed: 1 mixing bowl

4 egg yolks

2/3 cup olive oil

2/3 cup coconut oil

1 tbsp lemon juice

1 tsp Dijon mustard

Salt and black pepper

1. Whisk egg yolks together until smooth.
2. Add in lemon juice, spices, and mustard. Thoroughly combine.
3. Carefully add in the oils while whisking, starting with the olive oil. Only add in a drop of oil at a time, allowing it to fully emulsify before you continue pouring. Once the olive oil has been slowly added, do the same with the coconut oil.
4. Refrigerate, and then serve, or use as needed for up to one week.

Nutrition Facts (per serving):

Calories 131   Fat 14.9g

Carbs .2g   Protein .6g

Fight Yeast Infections

Again, coconut oil is great for killing bacteria. Simply apply, as a topical cream, to the infected area up to three times daily, and watch as your infection clears.

Sunscreen

Coconut oil has a natural SPF of 4. Stay safe from those harmful rays with this recipe for homemade sunscreen:

Simple Sunscreen

1/2 cup olive oil

1/4 cup coconut oil

2 tbsp zinc oxide

2 tbsp shea butter

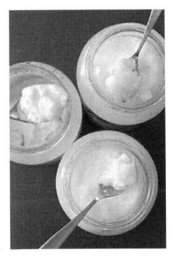

1. In a large glass jar, combine all ingredients except the zinc oxide. Put a lid on the jar.
2. Add a couple inches of water to a medium-sized saucepan. Place over medium heat.

3. Put the closed jar of ingredients in the heated water, and they will start to melt. Shake the jar occasionally to mix the ingredients better.

4. Once the ingredients have totally melted down, add in the zinc oxide, and stir well. Pour into a container of your choosing.

This recipe makes about a 25 SPF sunscreen. Best used within six months.

Energy Boost

Having a rough morning where all you want to do is crawl back into bed? Try taking one tablespoon of coconut oil with one tablespoon of chia seeds to perk you up and keep you going throughout the whole day.

Veins

Embarrassed by varicose or spider veins? Apply coconut oil regularly can help limit the appearance of both of these.

Arthritis

Due to coconut oil's anti-inflammatory properties, regularly applying a bit to arthritis-infected areas can help ease pain.

Mosquito Bites, Poison Ivy, and Chicken Pox

Itching like crazy? Apply coconut oil to the affected area to help sooth that irritating, insatiable burn.

Leather Softener

Rubbing just a small amount of coconut oil over shiny leather can help with its softness. Make sure the leather you want to use coconut oil on is shiny, though, or else it will disturb the look and feel of a more matte leather.

Throat Soother

When melted in with a hot cup of tea, coconut oil can help ease throat pain.

Vapor Rub

Can't beat that cold? Try this homemade vapor rub recipe, and get rid of coughing and congestion.

Vanquishing Vapor Rub

1/2 cup coconut oil

2 tbsp beeswax

3/4 tbsp eucalyptus oil

3/4 tbsp peppermint oil

1/2 tsp rosemary oil

1/2 tsp cinnamon oil

1. In a double broiler, melt the beeswax and coconut oil until just melted.
2. Add into the other oils. Stir until mixed well. Store in a sealable container, and apply to the chest or right below the nose as needed.

Hemorrhoid Help

When applied regularly, coconut oil can help relieve the pain of hemorrhoids.

Cold Sores

Coconut oil, with its bacteria-fighting properties, will naturally help clear up cold sores when applied regularly.

Acne Awareness

Mix equal parts of coconut oil with nutmeg to make a paste. Apply regularly to areas of acne on the face, back, or arms. The anti-inflammatory qualities will help reduce redness and swelling.

Heartburn and Nausea Soother

When mixed with a hot cup of ginger tea, coconut oil can help alleviate heartburn and nausea symptoms.

Warm Up

Coconut oil can help you keep your body warm when you're feeling cold. It works to raise your heart rate and internal temperature in a safe way. Consume it plain, or mix it in with a hot beverage.

Conclusion

Coconut oil is today's most trending oil.

Rich with medium-chain fatty acids, coconut oil is able to aid weight loss, lower cholesterol, strengthen the immune system, slow the process of aging, reverse Alzheimer's disease, and support countless beauty techniques and practices.

Simply adding coconut oil into your daily life will support all of these terrific benefits.
Cook with it, put it in your coffee, put it on your skin and in your hair -- the possibilities with coconut oil are endless.

If you are tired of spending oodles of money on over-the-counter products and prescription drugs, coconut oil is here to aid you with many aggravating issues. Buy it at your local grocery or health food store, and watch your overall health improve!

Other Books By Green Hills Press

Available on Kindle and in paperback on Amazon:

The Paleo Kitchen Series

*Paleo Bacon Cookbook: Lose Weight * Get Healthy * Eat Bacon*

Paleo Cravings: Your Favorite Comfort Foods Made Paleo

Paleo Easter Cookbook: Fast and Easy Recipes for Busy Moms

Paleo Party Food Cookbook: Make Your Friends Love You With Delicious & Healthy Party Food!

Paleo Pizza Cookbook: Lose Weight and Get Healthy by Eating the Food You Love

Paleo Valentine's Day Cookbook: Quick, Easy Recipes That Will Melt Your Lover's Heart

Simple Easy Paleo: Fast Fabulous Paleo Recipes with 5 Ingredients or Less

Please go to http://paleokindlebooks.com for more information.

TV and Movie Books

Call The Midwife!: Your Backstage Pass to the Era and the Making of the PBS TV Series

Doctor Who: 200 Facts on the Characters and Making of the BBC TV Series

Downton Abbey: Your Backstage Pass to the Era and Making of the TV Series

Sherlock Lives! 100+ Facts on Sherlock and the Smash Hit BBC TV Series

Other Books

KATE: Loyal Wife, Royal Mother, Queen-In-Waiting

HARRY: Popstar Prince

One Direction: Your Backstage Pass To The Boys, The Band, And The 1D Phenomenon

Find out more about these books at http://fandomkindlebooks.com.

Don't delay! Check them out today!

Coconut Health Made Simple

51041841R00046

Made in the USA
Lexington, KY
09 April 2016